The Birth Plan

SAMSARAH MORGAN

ISBN-13: 978-1543135053
ISBN-10: 1543135056

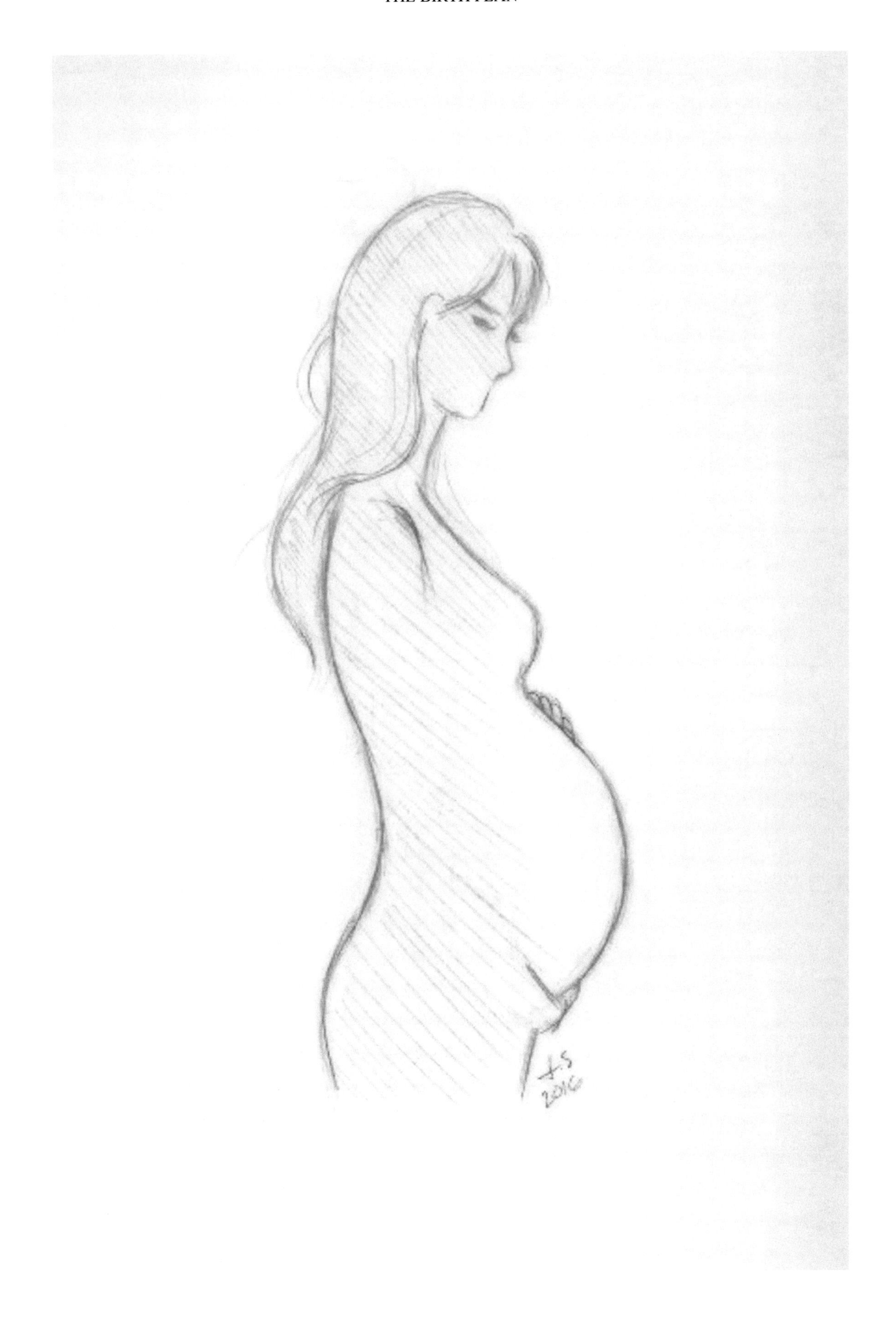

Dedication

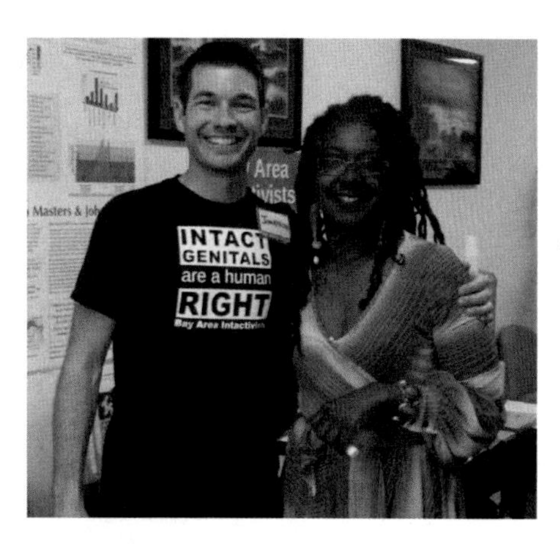

This little book, I dedicate to my dear friend Jonathon Conte. Jonathon was a tireless fighter for the genital integrity of children. He educated and warned of the harmful effects of male and female circumcision.

Jonathon died by his own hand. He died estranged from his family whom he felt were unable to empathize with the impact being circumcised, and it's meaning in his life and his connection to himself as a man.

My hope is that Jonathon has found peace and that now he is able to have a deep understanding of his goodness and how deeply he was loved by his devoted partner and his family of choice in the Bay Area Intactivist community.

Parents have so many choices to make. From the second they become aware of a pregnancy, until their young one steps out into the world as an adult. It's a daunting and often lonely task, for which many of us feel unprepared and sure are unsupported.

If I may offer a word of advice here, do your very best. Don't give up or in to "authority" figures and do your own in depth research; pro or con no matter the issue. Follow your gut - not your fear. At the end of the day, this is the best that any of us can do. Your decisions will have primary impact upon your child's ability to be a happy, healthy, self-assured human being: a friend, a lover, a co-worker, a mate, a parent to children of their own...

I believe that this is one of the deepest obligations we have as parents to do our best and then more than our best. And at the same time know that even when we do proceed with caution and education, not all of our decisions will impact our child as we wished.

Should that happen, I wish you the courage to hear your child's experience and reality. The courage to listen and offer love and an apology. Listen and refrain from defensiveness and have the courage to maintain an open door, through which your child can always find you waiting, full of love for them, on the other side.

May there be Peace in our hearts, homes, and our communities,
Samsarah Morgan, DD Cht. CD (ICTC) LC

If you would like to know more about intactivism please visit: www.bayareaintactivists.org and watch: *The Elephant in the Hospital: a discussion of circumcision.* https://youtu.be/oCEl4HphL9Y

Contents

FORWARD BY TANEFER CAMARA

From the moment one begins to even think of conception, there is not a moment too soon to start planning for your birth. Preparation for childbirth is more than just breathing techniques it is rather the ment and physical preparation for starting your family. You will explore the process of labor, birth and the postpartum period. You will also become familiar with common interventions, drugs and tools that aid, augment or induce labor and birth.

Having a birth plan means that you have explored the implications and possibilities of birth in either, home birth center or hospital and you have gained some knowledge about the birthing process and what that entails in various settings. You have chosen to becoming fully educated about this wonderful journey you and your family will soon embark upon.

A good birth plan is one that is well informed, thoughtful and cognizant of the unpredictable nature of childbirth. Your desire for a natural birth is based on the premise that birth is a natural physiological process and may be achieved with the right birthing team and in the right setting for your family. Planning your birth begins with imagining the possibility to bringing forth life in the most peaceful and gentle way possible. You may visualize the moment you touch your new baby for the first time and the first time your newborn suckles at your breast. Your plan is your guide when you are overwhelmed with intense sensations and emotions. It is also for your care team so that they may carry out your desires when possible and in the best interest of your and baby's health. Your plan challenges you to think about what to do if complications or crisis arise.

Planning your birth is about having an inner standing of yourself, your strength, your partner and family dynamics. The birth plan is designed with the goal of a healthy mother and baby in mind while simultaneously keeping your spiritual, cultural and familial beliefs and customs in alignment.

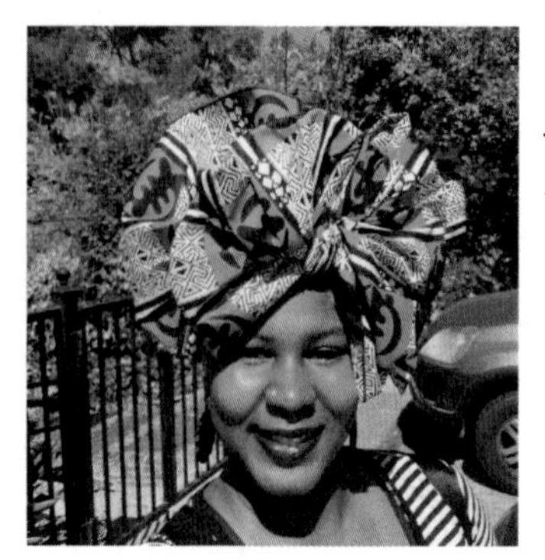

Samsarah Morgan has provided and helpful guide to get you started as you research and create your birth plan. I hope you enjoy its pages and share its information with other pregnant families. Enjoy this book and please enjoy your pregnancy!

TaNefer Camara, IBCLC
Watch *Teach Me How to Breastfeed* Video by TaNefer Camara
https://www.youtube.com/watch?v=HJVpzKi5pdo

Forward by Laura Marina Perez

Birth Plans

As an aspiring doula, I heard about the concept of the birth plans for the first time back in 1999. The idea was to give documentation to a laboring and birthing mama to present to the hospital staff so she could communicate what her desires and goals were for the birth of her baby. This made sense to me.

Now, as a practicing home birth midwife, I have a different relationship and understanding of birth plans. Some call them "birth preferences" in order to acknowledge that one cannot actually "plan" for a birth because no one knows how labor will begin or proceed; no one knows exactly what path a baby will take for her or his emergence.

Because I provide direct primary care for women and families deciding to birth outside of a hospital setting, I have intimate knowledge of their priorities, their expectations and even their fears about their upcoming birth journey. My clients don't need to develop a birth plan for their birth with me because we are able to discuss in detail what the process will likely be. However, I do ask my clients to create a birth plan in case of a non-emergent transfer to a hospital. In the unlikely scenario of transporting to a hospital, the birth plan is a useful tool to let nurses, residents, nurse-midwives, obstetricians and pediatricians know what the mama and her partner know about their choices for this life-changing event.

So, for those mamas and families planning to birth in the hospital, please know that you are deserving of full informed consent. This means getting information about a procedure or medication, their benefits and risks, their alternatives and what happens if the procedure or medication isn't used. You have the right to discuss your options with your partner and/or doula or midwife in private, if the situation isn't an emergency. I encourage all families to do their research (wherever you plan to birth!) so that you can truly make an informed choice about an intervention that presents itself to you. The birth plan is that documentation that expresses which interventions you will agree to and which you will decline, if at all possible.

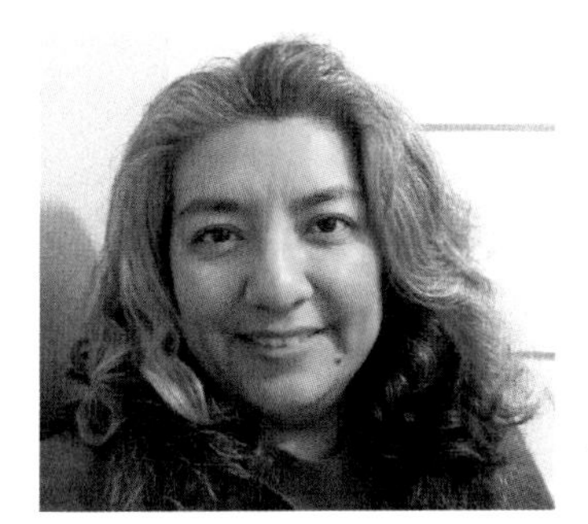

I truly hope that one day in the near future that every woman who wants a midwife and an out-of-hospital birth, will be able to access this care that respects their autonomy, their bodies, their babies and their families' values. Perhaps, then, birth plans will be obsolete and rarely used except in those cases when one needs to birth in a hospital, by medical necessity or choice.

Laura Marina Perez, CPM, LM
San Francisco, CA

A goal without a plan is just a wish.
Antoine de Saint Exupery.

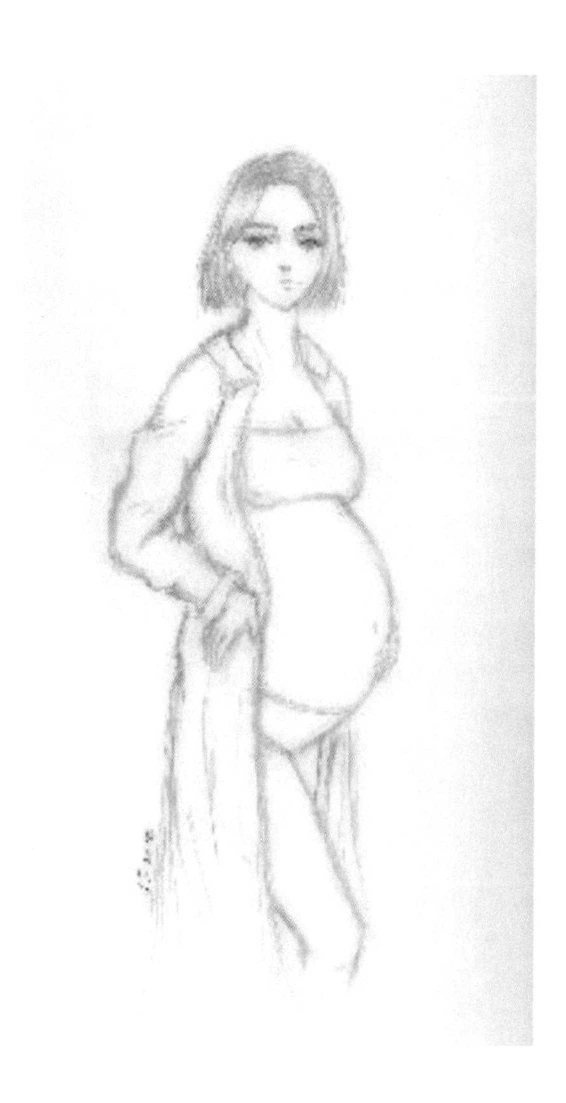

1 Introduction

As a birth doula, I have had the honor of assisting many families as they prepared for the births of their children. Whether you plan to have your child at home, free standing birth center or hospital, it is my belief that it is important for you to not just walk into this precious experience without preparation and planning.

A doula is a person who is acquainted and/or educated on the appropriate expectations in a natural birth. Your doula will work with you, filling in any holes in your research, providing any further referrals your family might need.

Planning means:

- ❑ Reading and educating yourself on pregnancy, labor, childbirth, breastfeeding and newborn care.
- ❑ Hire a doula, to be your educator, coach, and knowledgable friend.
- ❑ Take a childbirth education from an independent childbirth educator.
- ❑ Write a birth plan.

Many times my clients have told me that their OB has asked them - why they felt the need to prepare a plan. Birth is not linear they say - there are so many variables. How do you plan for it? Go with the flow they are told… Be open minded…

That thought process has always confused and amazed me. Do we tell our young people. "Why do you need to plan for your life? Why declare a major in college - why have a financial budget, just go with the flow - be flexible." Do we? Of course we don't that would be misguided and potentially dangerous advice.

Why is it that in birth, families are encouraged to set their intelligence and self determination aside and hand themselves over to the winds of fate? While it is true that there is an element of uncertainty in all of life, there is a great deal that a healthy expectant mother can expect and plan for in her pregnancy and birth process.

She is a an expectant mother not an uncertain mother. She expects - not guesses.

- ❑ Generally a couple sits down to write the birth plan in their third trimester.
- ❑ Optimally, they have taken childbirth education and preparation classes.
- ❑ Educate yourself fully pro and con on all of the various childbirth and early parenting controversies, such as vaccination, medicated vs. non-medicated birth, breastfeeding vs. exclusive bottle feeding, circumcision - I will provide a few resources in this book - but don't stop there. Get all the information you can to fuel the best decisions for your family.
- ❑ Also extremely important are breastfeeding and newborn care classes to be prepared for the first and crucial first few months as the parent of a newborn.

- ❑ Hopefully they have been under the care of a midwife or obstetrician who has aware of their needs and desire for a natural childbirth or for a birth that omits certain interventions.

- ❑ It is vital that all options be clearly discussed with your healthcare provider to be sure that your midwife or OB is on board with your birth vision.

- ❑ Tour the hospital or birth center in which you plan to deliver your child.

- ❑ Discuss with the tour guide what your wishes and plans are for your birth.

- ❑ Ask the hospital about its C-section rate.

- ❑ Ask your birthing center or home birth midwife about their transport rate find out why and under what circumstances transports are done.

All of this research and preparation helps a family to solidify their vision. It may also mean that you have made the choice to change health care personnel who seemed reluctant to answer your questions or those whose answers were vague or disrespectful.

All of this may seem a great deal of work. And it may prove to be - but isn't it worth it? You would have done all you can - by your own clear thinking, pointed questions, and self care to align yourself with nature. Nature wants babies; wants them healthy and in the arms of healthy mothers and adoring partners. Wants them welcomed into devoted communities, family groups and extended family groups who are waiting to support the families as they raise up a new generation.

Imagine that as you do all the right eating exercising, reading, questioning - imagine your healthy and vital newborn child. Imagine yourself connected, excited and confident. Once you have gathered all your information. You can sit down with either with your doula to discuss how she/he will walk with you on your birth journey.

I usually recommend that my clients create two plans: One for momma (birthing person) and one for baby. This is particularly helpful in the hospital setting as there will be two departments who will be responsible for the care of momma and baby: obstetrics and pediatrics.

Obstetrics usually doesn't need to know that you wish to opt out of the antibiotic eye ointment for your newborn. Similarly, pediatrics does not need to know that you do wish soft lighting while you labor. On a similar vein, your OB doesn't need to know that you want Enya playing as you labor - but your doula does - as she will be the one keeping the CD or Ipod playing for you!

Your birth plan gives everyone on your birth team a clear understanding of your wishes and expectations during your labor and birth. It allows your family and other helpers to provide the best possible support for your birth as possible. At the end of this process, what you will emerge with will be a two page document.

The first page focuses on the wishes and desires of the birthing person — during labor — usually broken down by stage:

- Early labor
- active labor
- transition
- pushing and delivery of the baby
- delivery of the placenta

The baby's plan will discuss which newborn procedures are being declined and informing the hospital staff to provide you with the necessary form to decline such procedures. Baby's plan will state as well your plans to breastfeed your baby, and desire that your child not be offered formula, or a pacifier as you are wanting to create a strong breastfeeding bond with your child.

- ❑ Your completed plan should be reviewed with your doctor or midwife and a copy of it should be placed in your chart.

- ❑ Your doula should carry 3-5 copies of it in her file for you and bring them with her to your birth.

- ❑ Your doula will provide one of the birth plans to the nurse in triage at the hospital and be sure that th nurses who will support you during your labor and throughout shift changes are aware and have seen the plan.

- ❑ I recommend placing a copy of the baby's plan on the warming table in your hospital room. This ensures that the pediatric staff will see and respond to it.

- ❑ Remember, that when you signed into the hospital, you signed permissions for the staff to do all that they deem necessary for your care and that of your child. If you decline one of these interventions, yo must sign a waiver stating that you take responsibility for this choice and no not wish a particular intervention. You may have to sign a form for each intervention you decline. Don't let this surprise you…

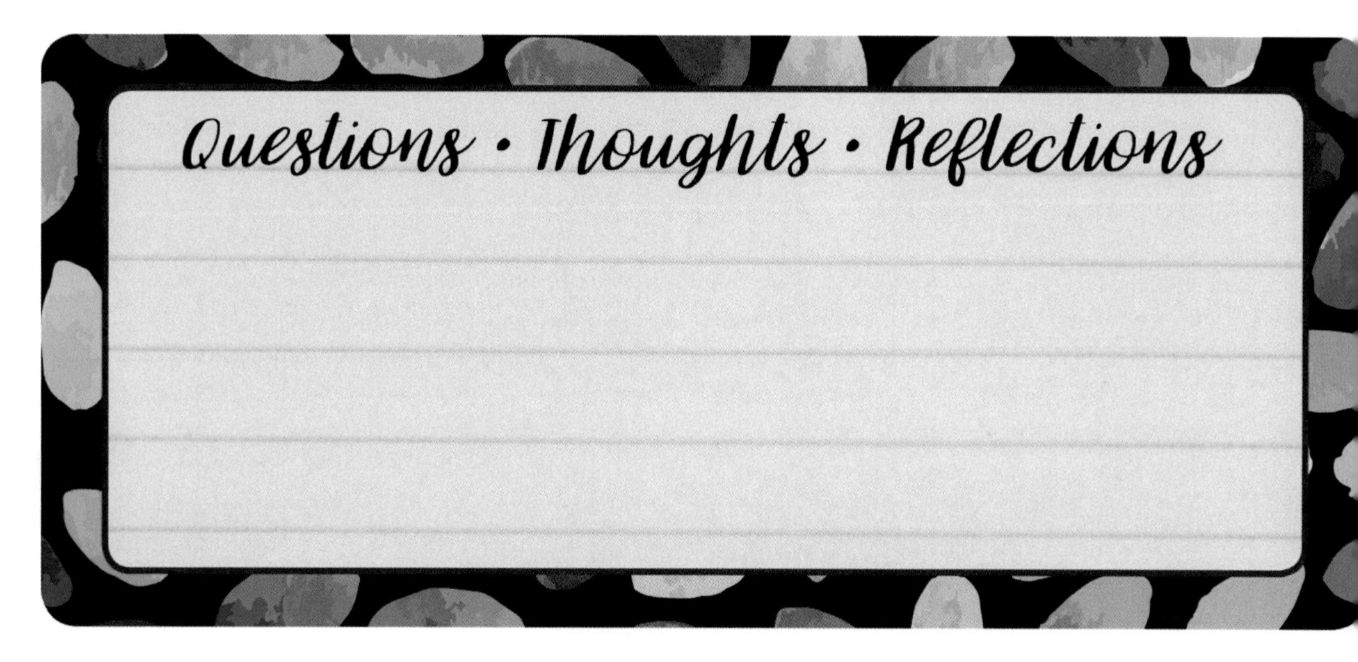

2 A Word About Pain Medications

My first suggestion is to let your doula be your pain killer. Pick a doula with whom you feel trust and allow her to offer you the many tools she has to support you through labor. For the majority of birthing people - this is all you will to be able to birth without medications.

There are also very sound reasons where pain medications can be strategically used to maybe help a mom get some rest and be able to have a vaginal birth rather than a C-section (Cesarean section).

Discuss all of these options fully and make the decision that feels right in your mind and body for your baby and circumstances.

Be aware of all of the possible side effects of any medications offered and be prepared to address them after the birth of your child to assist detox and recovery from the needed medications.

Acquaint yourself with the alternative health care providers who may be of tremendous support after your birth (and also during pregnancy) i.e. chiropractic, naturopath, acupuncturist, acupressurist, herbalist. Be sure to work with certified or licensed holistic health practitioners who have experience in supporting pregnant bodies and babies…

There is no shame or mistake in taking a necessary drug. All things have their place and time.

3 A Word About C-sections

I have also heard it said that it makes no sense to plan because if you "end up with a C-section" you will feel disappointed. Let me say that a needed C-section is not a lesser form of birth. If you are one of the 1 per cent of birthing mothers who experience a true emergency, rather than disappointment, let's be at peace that medical intervention was there when you needed it. And sure you may feel disappointment but I hope that that disappointment will be soothed by the knowledge that you did all you could for your baby, including receiving life saving surgery.

Feel your feelings, get support, love yourself and adore your baby… You have not failed - you've won the best, sweetest and most challenging of prizes, you or you and your partner have a newborn to raise!

If your C-section is due to a true emergency, it can be a loving and family centered event. Talk to your doctor and hospital, and add to your birth plan you desire for: photos, music and skin to skin with your newborn as soon as possible under your circumstance. Breastfeeding should be initiated as soon as reasonably possible to aid recovery for both you and your baby.

4 Controversies

Building your birth plan is an exercise in doing what you will have to do several million times as a parent - and that is making sometime difficult and controversial decisions. When I was an eighteen year old mother and I decided that I wanted a natural birth of my twin sons and then to breastfeed my children - many people thought that I was crazy! A few even thought that they should warn me that I was putting myself and my children at risk! I had to stand strong and have faith in the research I had done and the support team that I'd gathered around and ultimately faith in my own body that I could have my babies as I envisioned - and I did.

The following are some controversial topics to consider and add to your birth plan. Please take the time with your partner and support system to research these procedures and know that you have the right to choose or refuse any of them.

My job here is to not give you my opinion. Only to lay out the particulars. You and you alone are the parent of your child. Your responsibility is to do your own research pro or con on each issue, and then to make your own best decision as a single parent or couple. Let a vision of your child as a happy healthy adult be your guide.

5 Immunizations & Injectables

For your birth plan - there are only two immunizations or injected supports that might be offered to you those are for: Hepatitis B and Vitamin K and a flu shot.

Hepatitis B is a disease contracted by IV drug use or by having sex with someone who has it. It is the firs immunization offered to US babies and will be administered within the first 24 hours unless that parent refuses it.

Vitamin K is administered due to a concern that the newborn liver might not be able to perform the processes needed to clot blood. This might be because mothers have not consumed the raw ingredients necessary to have a good enough stores of Vitamin K in their infant's body after birth. Vitamin K is found in abundance in green leafy vegetables. If the mother has maintained a balanced diet with and abundance of Vitamin K on board - there will be plenty to have shared with her baby and to be present in her colostrum (the baby's first food) and her milk supply.

Vitamin K is also available in a liquid form, so if a family decides that they wish to have extra vitamin k that will probably have to be requested in advance from the hospital as it is usually not on hand. I challenge that I have heard of is that the baby can have a negative reaction to the taste of the liquid supplement, and tha this reaction can interfere with early breastfeeding and bonding.

Flu shots and Hep B

Many mothers are being offered a flu shot during their pregnancies. Some hospitals are offering flu shots to newborn before they leave the hospital. You have the right to refuse this, or to wait to have the shots given by your pediatrician, or not give the shot at all.

Some parents have concerns regarding the additives, preservatives, and ingredients found in these and other immunizations and shots, they feel that these ingredients might cause health concerns in the future for their child.

Some parents would simply like to not administer vaccines and other shots on the very first day of their child's life. They might want to wait to do more research and or discuss the matter with their pediatrician.

Again, this is your baby, and your decision, and if you say no to any of these in the hospital, be prepared to sign a release form, and be prepared to have the hospital pediatrics staff speak to you with regard to your decision. They are looking at these decision from a public health standpoint and are offering you what they have been trained see as the best road for your family to take.

If you live in the state of California, the new vaccine law SB277 mandates vaccines per the CDC schedule if your child is going to daycare or public or private school. Only home schooled children are exempt from this requirement, and those who have been given a medical exemption from a qualified medical health professional. Please carefully read and understand this law - to assist you here is the entire text of this law. https://leginfo.legislature.ca.gov/faces/billNavClient.xhtml?bill_id=201520160SB277

Researching Vaccines

The CDC website provides up to date information on our government health's official opinion on the effectiveness and scheduling of vaccines for US children. This information and these guidelines are the ones followed by pediatricians. Their website is http://www.cdc.gov/

There are many books written to discuss reported concerns with vaccines and possible alternative schedules for the administration of vaccines. Some are: *The Vaccine Book* by Dr. Robert Sears, *Vaccine Epidemic: How Corporate Greed, Biased Science, and Coercive Government Threaten Our Human Rights, Our Health, and Our Children* by Louise Kuo Habakus, Mary Holland and *Dissolving Illusions: Disease Vaccines and Forgotten History* by Dr Suzanne Humphries, MD.

6 Bathing the Baby

Your newly born baby isn't dirty.

The inside of your womb is a sterile cavity. We humans, like other mammals have a need to hold, smell, touch, and taste our offspring, and they have the same desire to bond with us. Bathing actually washes away very important biochemical information and is wholly unnecessary.

Some babies a born with a coating of creamy substance called vernix. This substance kept your little one from puckering up in your womb. Feel free to rub it into your little ones skin, it's the finest lotion ever conceived and is not DIRT!

Take a whiff! You and your partner will never experience anything that smells as wonderful as your newborn baby. When you are home and settled, your doula or maybe a grandma, can help you to give your little one its first bath. Please continue to use scent free soaps to avoid exposure to toxic chemicals and, this goes for Momma too - your smell is helping your baby to connect with you, bond and love you. Your ability to smell each other's natural scent aids healing and assists breastfeeding and bonding - take a whiff!

7 Circumcision

Is the removal of the foreskin of a baby boy's foreskin (the skin covering the head of the penis). Many parents are now opting not to circumcise their sons, and the American Pediatric Association has stated that there isn't enough benefit to the operation to make it a routine event for newborn boys. It's is more and more simply being considered a cosmetic operation, and there are health plans that will not cover it for that reason.

There are religious customs that call for circumcision, and in that case the family would meet with their clergy on the seventh day of life to perform the religious ceremony. It's not surprising to me that that day is the when most babies bodies are manufacturing the clotting factor needed to prevent hemorrhage. The religious ceremony for Jewish families is called a Bris. There is a movement within reform communities of Jewish families to allow for a ceremony that provides the rich religious significance of a Bris without cutting - this ceremony is called a Brit Shalom visit this link to find out more about hsi option. http://www.britshalom.info/ And a very beautiful book on this topic is *Celebrating Brit Shalom* by Rebecca Wald.

8 Co-Sleeping / Family Bedding

The following is totally my opinion. Since the dawn of time human beings have slept with their newborns and young children. There I said it!

There is a great deal of concern regarding family bedding and there are pediatricians who actively seek to discourage it. I certainly agree that there are safe ways to share a family bed and ways that might be problematic. This all depends on your baby, family and circumstances. However, in the first few weeks being very close and possibly skin to skin with your newborn is a very helpful tool in: maintaining bonding, easier and efficient breastfeeding, and ensuring more rest, since baby can be fed while side lying rather than sitting up in a chair, propped up with pillows.

What follows are links to more information of co sleeping, attachment parenting as well as the APA American Pediatric Association's Statement on Co Sleeping.
https://www.aap.org/en-us/about-the-aap/aap-press-room/pages/AAP-Expands-Guidelines-for-Infant-Sleep-Safety-and-SIDS-Risk-Reduction.aspx

Bed Sharing with baby the risks and benefits, from Medical News Today
http://www.medicalnewstoday.com/articles/284275.php

Ensure safe sleep - an article from Attachment Parenting International
http://www.attachmentparenting.org/principles/night

Sleeping with your baby. A parent's guide to co-sleeping by James McKenna Phd.
A Quick Guide to Safely Sleeping With Your Baby by James McKenna Phd.

Once again - educate yourself fully and make the best decision for: baby, family and situation. Your baby needs access to your body, your body needs to hold your baby close, and excellent book on the challenges of our culture is *Nighttime Breastfeeding: An American Cultural Dilemma* by Cecilia Tomari.

9 CONGRATULATIONS!

Your plan now is:

- ❑ written
- ❑ discussed
- ❑ may be edited
- ❑ and now rests in your doula's hands
- ❑ and in your midwife or doctor's charts for you

Thank you for this vital gift you have given your baby and yourself… All of these classes, this preparation and the additional staffing up will pay off. And now, you are ready to wait with grace and courage into the great mystery of birth! You have done your part, you have taken care of your body, you have set your intention and NOW you can let go! Let go and give yourself to birth, lose yourself to find yourself in the specific rhythm and flow of what your labor will mean for you. This rhythm will be unique to you, your baby, your relationship, your world. You are not a product on a conveyor belt, you are not a cookie cutter pressing out an experience identical to others.

You are a unique human consciousness bringing another unique human consciousness into this world. You are powerful beyond imagining. You have prepared mind, body and soul for this moment. And you can do this! Your partner, your family, your medical or midwifery staff and your doula all stand waiting to support you, as you powerfully guide your little one out of your body and into your arms.

You got this!
You got this momma!
Brava!

And if there is anyway I can support you, please let me know!

10 A Word about Doulas

Doulas are an incredibly helpful part of any family's birth team. Please do not let finances keep you from receiving their support! Many doulas offer a sliding scale fee offering care to all families regardless of their ability to pay.

Talk to your doula, it is sometimes possible to have your doula fee reimbursed to you by your insurance company (PPOs only). Some hospitals have volunteer doula programs that offer free services to families in need.

Finding a doula:

- ICTC - International Center for Traditional Childbearing www.ictcmidwives,org
- DONA - Doulas of North America www.dona.org
- CAPPA - Childbirth and Postpartum Professional Organization www.cappa.net
- Oakland Better Birth Foundation (San Francisco Bay Area Doulas) www.oaklandbetterbirthfoundation.com

11 Suggested Reading List

A Thinking Woman's Guide To a Better Birth by Henci Goer

The Doula Guide to Birth by Lowe and Zimmerman

Ina Mae's Guide to Birth by Ina Mae Gaskin

Birthing Justice: Black Women Pregnancy and Childbirth by Oparah and Bonneparte

Birth: A Black Woman's Survival Guide by Samsarah Morgan (when released)

References

The Earth Momma Blog Free Birth Plan
http://blog.earthmamaangelbaby.com/birth-plan/

The Birth Plan Your Expectations And Preferences
http://www.babycenter.com/calculators-birthplan

The Birth Book by Sears and Sears

The Doula Guide To Childbirth by Lowe and Zimmerman

About the Contributors

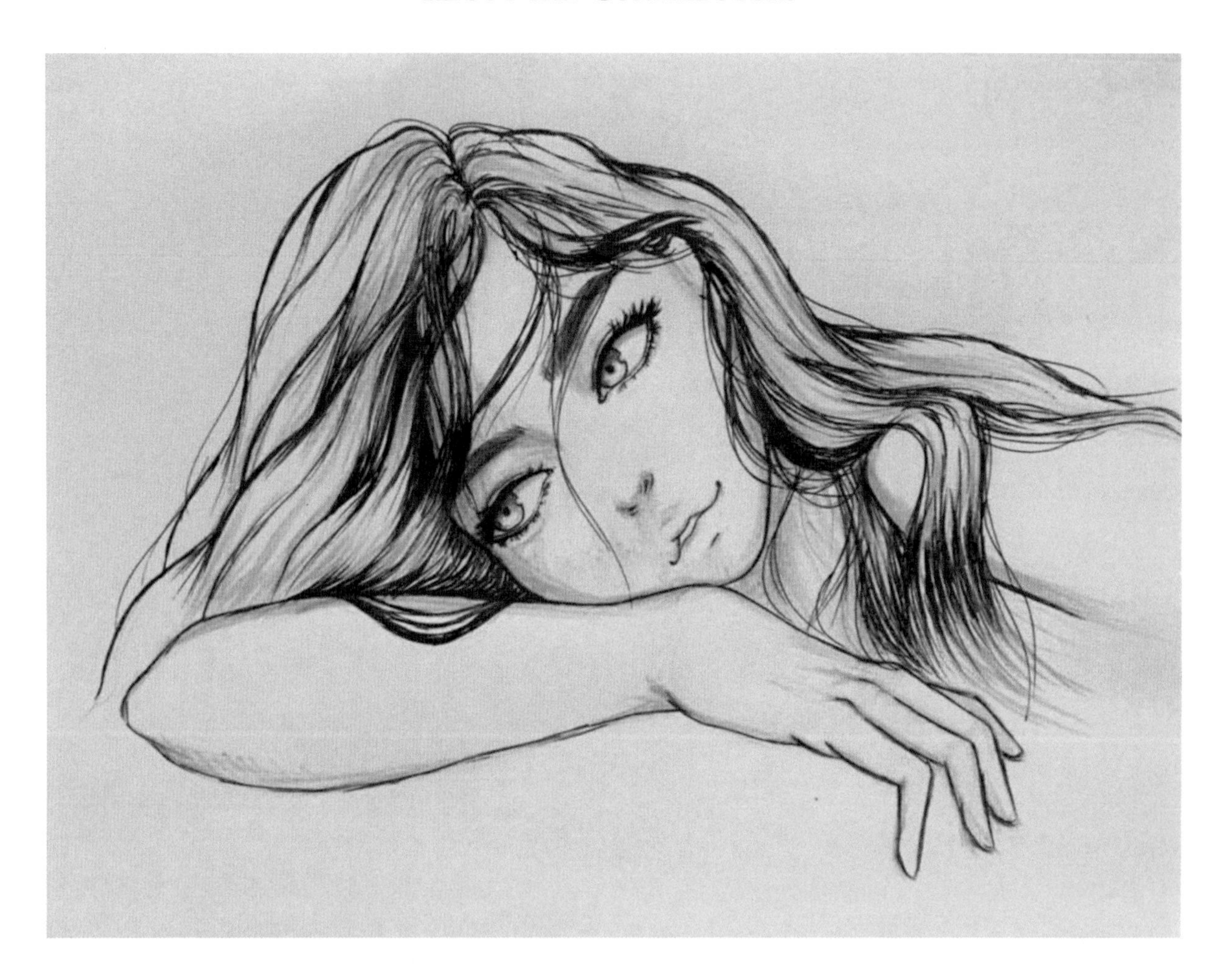

Jazmine A. Silver (illustrations) is an illustrator and computer artist in Oakland, CA. She is a student at Oakland Technical High School. She loves drawing, math, music, her dog Django, her younger brother Gio, and Ferrero Rocher chocolates. She has been a fine artist since toddlerhood. She is the Granddaughter of the author and her artwork was featured in Samsarah Morgan's first book *Children's Village Tales of an Urban Nana.* Other samples of her work can be seen on her **Instagram account @jazmo.art**

Lita Mikrut (cover design / layout) "I am a digital doula and graphic designer providing creative marketing services for print and web. Specializing in working with individuals; with an expertise in working with Community Groups, Fine Arts, Healing Arts, and Family/Children's Organizations. I trained to be a birth doula under Samsarah's loving teachings and wisdoms. I also had the special experience of working with Samsarah as my doula, at my daughter's birth. With gratitude, I was able to share in the creation of this book along with Samsarah. May it serve well — the good health and circle of family." litamikrut.com

Syan de LuMargh-Jones (copy-editor) is a virtual assistant, researcher, writer, and copy-editor. She is also a wellness facilitator and life coach with over fifteen years experience working with groups and individuals helping them to breath life into their deepest desires and take action to live the life of their dreams. 5thelementmedicine@gmail.com

About the Author

Samsarah Morgan is a birth and postpartum doula, childbirth, breastfeeding and parenting educator. She is a bereavement counselor and doula. She is an interfaith minister counselor, hypnotherapist and family life coach. Fall 2016, she celebrated thirty-seven years as a birthworker.

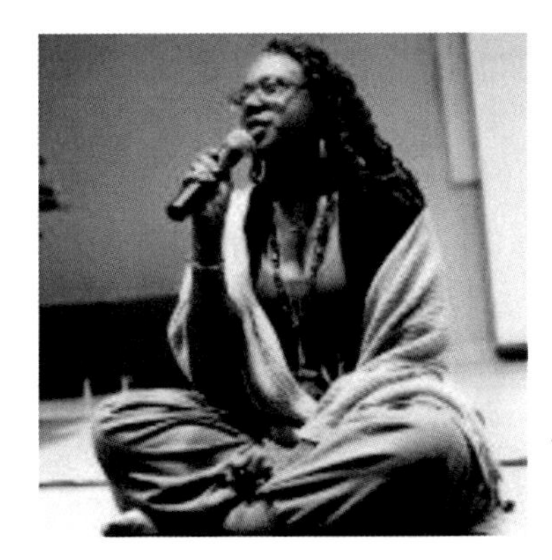

She is the Founder and Executive Director of *Oakland Better Birth Foundation.* She is Founder and Director of *Nia Healing Center for Birth and Family Life*, *Shiphrah's Circle Community Doula Program*, *Birth Professionals of America* and *Bay Area Birth Keeper Doulas.*

Samsarah has trained doulas under her own organization for twenty years and is an certified trainer for an *ICTC International Center for Traditional Childbearing, full circle doula certification program.*

Other Books by this Author

Samsarah Morgan is the Author of:

- *Children's Village Tales of An Urban Nana* (2015)
- *The Birth Plan* (2017)
- *Birth: A Black Woman's Survival Guide* (expected due date 2017)

Connect with Samsarah Morgan

Please feel free to reach out to Samsarah with questions, requests for speaking engagements, or to inquire about training opportunities and services by **calling 510-496-3491, or by email lsamsarahmorgan@gmail.com or nia.healing.center@gmail.com**

visit the websites
www.niahealingcenter.org
www.oaklandbetterbirthfoundation.com
www.doulasamsarah.wordpress.com

Find her on Facebook:
Nia Healing Center for Birth and Family Life
https://www.facebook.com/Niafamilylifecenter/
Oakland Better Birth Foundation
https://www.facebook.com/4allbabiesbetterbirths
Samsarah Morgan
https://www.facebook.com/doulasamsarah

Questions • Thoughts • Reflections

THE Birth Plan

{Mother / Birthing Person's Full Name} {Today's Date}

{Father / Partner's Full Name} {Due Date}

HomeBirth & Hospital Birth Options Checklist - page 1 of 2

Attendents & Amenities:

I'd like the following people to be present during labor and/or birth:

- ☐ *Partner:* ________________
- ☐ *Friends:* ________________
- ☐ *Relative/s:* ________________
- ☐ *Doula:* ________________
- ☐ *Children:* ________________

I'd also like:

- ☐ *To bring music.*
- ☐ *To dim the lights.*
- ☐ *To wear my own clothes during labor and delivery.*
- ☐ *To take pictures and/or recordings during labor and delivery.*

Labor:

- ☐ *I'd like the option of returning home if I'm not in active labor.*

If I'm admitted, I'd like:

- ☐ *My partner to be allowed to stay with me at all times.*
- ☐ *Only my practitioner, nurse, and guests present (i.e. no residents, medical students, or other hospital personnel).*
- ☐ *To wear my contact lenses, as long as I don't need a c-section.*
- ☐ *To eat if I wish to.*
- ☐ *To stay hydrated by drinking clear fluids instead of having an IV.*
- ☐ *To walk and move around as I choose.*

As long as the baby and I are doing fine, I'd like:

- ☐ *To have intermittent rather than continous electronic fetal monitoring.*
- ☐ *To be allowed to progress free of stringent time limits.*
- ☐ *Limited cervical check.*
- ☐ *Natural water rupture.*
- ☐ *To wear my own clothes during labor and delivery.*
- ☐ *To take pictures and/or recordings during labor and delivery.*

If they're available, I'd like to try:

- ☐ *A birthing stool.*
- ☐ *A birthing chair.*
- ☐ *A squatting bar.*
- ☐ *A birthing pool/tub.*

I'd like to bring the following equipment with me:

- ☐ *A birthing stool.*
- ☐ *A beanbag chair.*
- ☐ *A birthing pool/tub.*
- ☐ *Other:* ________________

When it's time to push, I'd like:

- ☐ *To do so instinctively.*
- ☐ *A warm compress (if not a water birth).*

NIA Healing Center
KNOWLEDGE LIBRARY
www.NiaHealingCenter.org

THE
Birth Plan

{Mother / Birthing Person's Full Name} {Today's Date}

{Father / Partner's Full Name} {Due Date}

HomeBirth & Hospital Birth Options Checklist - page 2 of 2

Pain Relief

I'd like to try the following pain-management techniques:

- [ ] Acupressure
- [ ] Bath /shower
- [ ] Hot / Cold therapy
- [ ] Self-hypnosis
- [ ] Massage
- [ ] Breathing techniques / distraction
- [ ] Please don't offer me pain medication. I'll request it if I need it.

Vaginal Birth

I'd like:

- [ ] To view the birth using a mirror.
- [ ] To touch my baby's head as it crowns.
- [ ] The room to be as quiet as possible.
- [ ] To risk a tear rather than have an episiotomy.
- [ ] My partner to 'catch' our baby.

Cesarean Section

If I have a c-section, I'd like:

- [ ] My partner present at all times during the operation and for my partner to 'catch' our baby.
- [ ] The screen lowered a bit so I can see my baby coming out.
- [ ] The baby given to my partner as soon as he's dried (as long as he's in good health).
- [ ] To breastfeed my baby in the recovery room.
- [ ] I would like my doula to accompany my partner and I during the operation, and to stay with me, should my child need to go the nursery for evaluation or tests.
- [ ] I would like to have skin to skin contact with my child as soon as possible and while c-section is being repaired.
- [ ] I would prefer to be repaired using stitches rather than staples.

After birth, I'd Like:

- [ ] To hold my baby right away, putting off any procedures that aren't urgent.
- [ ] To breastfeed as soon as possible.
- [ ] To wait until the umbilical cord stops pulsating before it's clamped and cut.
- [ ] My partner to cut the cord
- [ ] Not to get routine oxytocin (Pitocin) after I deliver the placenta.
- [ ] To take pictures and/or recordings during labor and delivery.

Postpartun

After delivery, I'd like:

- [ ] All newborn procedures to take place in my presence.
- [ ] My partner to stay with the baby at all times if I can't be there.
- [ ] To stay in a private room.
- [ ] To have a cot provided for my partner.
- [ ] My baby fed on demand. I plan to Breastfeed exclusively.
- [ ] Please don't offer anything to my baby at any point (e.g. sugar water, pacifer).
- [ ] My other children brought in to see us as soon as possible after the birth.
- [ ] 24hour rooming with my baby.
- [ ] I'm interested in checking out of the hospital early.

NIA Healing Center
KNOWLEDGE LIBRARY
www.NiaHealingCenter.org

THE
Birth Plan

{Mother / Birthing Person's Full Name} {Today's Date}

{Father / Partner's Full Name} {Due Date}

BIRTH and POSTPARTUM PLAN - Transporting

(mother) and (partner) have transferred to the hospital for their birth based upon unforeseen circumstances. (mother) and (partner) desire to be informed about any and all procedures before they are performed including what the procedure entails, the risks and benefits of the procedure, any alternatives to the procedure and what may occur if the procedure is not done. Thank you for respecting our wishes.

FOR LABOR:

- [ ] *(partner) is to be present with (mother) at all times.*
- [ ] *(mother) would like freedom of movement to be able to labor in any position she likes.*
- [ ] *We request a telemetry unit for fetal monitoring to assist with freedom of movement.*
- [ ] *Please do not offer (mother) any pain medication. She will request it, if she wants it.*
- [ ] *Please keep lights in the room at a dim setting.*
- [ ] *(mother) desires minimal intrusions.*
- [ ] *Student doctors and nurses are not welcome as a part of (mother)'s care.*
- [ ] *We do not consent to the use of a fetal scalp electrode unless medically indicated.*
- [ ] *(mother) does not consent to amniotomy as a labor induction method unless she understands and agrees that it is medically necessary.*
- [ ] *(mother) would like to follow her own pushing urges. This means no coached pushing.*

BIRTH & IMMEDIATE POSTPARTUM:

- [ ] *(mother) does not consent to an episiotomy.*
- [ ] *(partner) would like to catch the baby.*
- [ ] *There will be immediate skin-to-skin contact between baby and (mother) after baby is born.*
- [ ] *All newborn assessments are to be done while baby is with (mother).*
- [ ] *Please delay clamping and cutting of the umbilical cord until after it has stopped pulsing.*
- [ ] *(mother) does not consent to pitocin in the 3rd stage. She will use her own maternal effort to birth her placenta.*
- [ ] *(mother) plans on holding on to her placenta.*

IF CESAREAN SECTION OCCURS:

- [ ] *(mother) does not consent to general anesthesia.*
- [ ] *(mother)'s (partner) will be present with (mother) in the Operating Room.*
- [ ] *(partner) will stay with the baby at all times, including during the initial assessment of the baby and if the baby must be taken to the nursery.*
- [ ] *(mother) will have another support person with her in the OR if (partner) leaves with the baby.*
- [ ] *(mother) consents to antibiotics only after surgery.*
- [ ] *(mother) would like to have skin to skin contact with my child as soon as possible and while c-section is being repaired.*
- [ ] *(mother) would prefer to be repaired using stitches rather than staples.*

THE
Birth Plan

{Mother / Birthing Person's Full Name} {Today's Date}

{Father / Partner's Full Name} {Due Date}

BIRTH and POSTPARTUM PLAN for BABY - Transporting

We request that any procedures and assessments happen in the birth room with both parents present. If the baby is in need of any assessments in another location outside of the birth room, then (partner) will be with the baby at all times. Thank you for respecting our wishes.

POSTPARTUM and NEWBORN CARE:

- ☐ *Immediate skin-to-skin contact between (mother) and her baby.*
- ☐ *Baby will be rooming in with (mother).*
- ☐ *(mother) will be exclusively breastfeeding her baby. This means that we do not consent to giving the baby formula, glucose water or a pacifier.*
- ☐ *We do not consent to the Vitamin K injection.*
- ☐ *We do not consent to the erythromycin eye ointment.*
- ☐ *We do not want the baby to be bathed in the hospital.*
- ☐ *We do not consent to a circumcision being performed.*
- ☐ *We do not consent to the Newborn Screen. Our midwives will provide this service to us during our postpartum period.*

NIA
Healing Center
KNOWLEDGE LIBRARY
www.NiaHealingCenter.org

Made in the USA
Middletown, DE
21 September 2020